All-Natural Homemade Lip Balms

Total Lip Care Guide for Healthy Glowing Lips

Josephine Simon

Disclaimer and Terms of Use

Efforts have been made to ensure that the information in this book is accurate and complete. However, the author and the publisher do not warrant the accuracy of the information, text, and graphics contained within the book due to the rapidly changing nature of science, research, known and unknown facts, and internet. The author and the publisher do not hold any responsibility for errors, omissions, or contrary interpretation of the subject matter herein. This book is presented solely for motivational and informational purposes only. The publisher and author of this book does not control or direct users' actions and are not responsible for the information or content shared, harm and/or action of the book readers. The information herein is offered for informational purposes solely and is universal as so. The presentation of the information is without contract or any type of guarantee assurance.

ISBN: 9781675608890

Printed in the United States

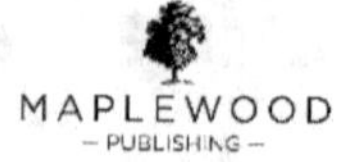

CONTENTS

LIP CARE

No matter where we go, our lips are constantly exposed to the elements. Heat, sun, and cold all present their challenges for the lips' delicate skin. We don't have oil glands in our lips, so they can dry out fast. We need to provide moisture and protection to keep our lips feeling and looking good.

Enter the beauty industry! Every year, millions of tubes and tubs of lip sticks, glosses, and balms are sold, and we all have our favorites. But did you know that many of the products you can buy contain ingredients that are bad for you? Some are designed to dry the lips so you'll reach for the product over and over throughout the day.

Well, the jig's up. It turns out that nature provides several healthy alternatives to the standard store-bought options, and you're likely to have some of them in your home already. We'll show you how to create safe and effective lip care products, including natural UV protectants and moisturizers.

We're so excited to share this collection of healthy lip treatments with you. We'll show you the tremendous variety of options you have, and our formulas include NO harmful ingredients.

We've gathered a selection of scrubs, like <u>Gingerbread Lip Scrub</u>, and <u>Plumping Coffee Lip Scrub</u>. Once you've exfoliated, you can apply one of our amazing lip masks, like <u>Cucumber Green Tea Lip Mask</u>, or our <u>Aloe Vera Overnight Mask</u>. And of course, we have some fun and nourishing balms to tell you about, like <u>Chocolate Mint Lip Balm</u> (which makes a great gift), <u>Goat's Milk Balm</u>, and <u>Party Swirl</u>!

All these recipes are inexpensive and easy to make. We think that once you start customizing and using your favorite blends, you won't miss the retail products. With this book, you can begin making and sharing lip care products that support your health with natural ingredients.

Many of us have a little addiction to lip balm that keeps us reaching for commercial products that contain a baffling list of ingredients – some of which are harmful. Here are some things you shouldn't be putting on your lips.

<u>Petroleum jelly</u>. We know your mother (and her mother) always reached for petroleum jelly as a cure-all for skin and lip ailments. And while it does have its uses, we don't suggest putting it on your mouth. Petrolatum (aka petroleum jelly or mineral oil) is processed from petroleum using toxic compounds. Since it's not meant to be ingested, there's a good chance it's tainted with contaminants from processing. Coconut oil makes a lovely substitute.

<u>Parabens</u>. The body may confuse parabens with estrogen. Parabens have been linked to breast cancer and melanomas as well as reduced testosterone levels in men. Obviously, it's best to avoid these.

<u>BHA and BHT</u>. These chemicals (butylated hydroxyanisole and butylated hydroxytoluene) are used as preservatives, but your body won't like them. They can interfere with your hormones and cause cancer, birth defects, and developmental disorders.

<u>Flavors and Fragrances</u>. These are chemical compounds that often contain high levels of phthalates. These are more ingredients that are shown to interfere with the body's natural systems, disrupting hormones and causing allergy symptoms as well as reduced fertility for everyone.

So, do we have your attention? Let's not hand our money over to companies who don't seem to be keeping our best interests in mind. Read on to learn how to cut these products out of your life and replace them with lip treatments known to support your health.

Lip Care in Summer and Winter

Rain or shine, your lips need care to keep them healthy and looking great. Here is how you go about it.

Summer Lip Care Tips

- Treat your lips with coconut oil every day. Massage the oil gently onto your lips and leave it to be absorbed.
- Eat balanced food that keeps your body hydrated.
- Increase your water intake. Drink lots of healthy juices.
- Apply lip balm to save your lips from exposure to the sun.
- Exfoliate your lips twice a week using a lip scrub or any other gentle method.
- Apply coconut oil to your lips before going to bed.

Winter Lip Care Tips

- Exfoliate your lips once or twice a week with a lip scrub.
- Apply natural oils for moisturizing your lips.
- Apply butter to your lips.
- Massage your lips with ointment-based lip balm before sleep to prevent dryness.
- Avoid licking your lips.
- Do not scrub your lips when they are flaky.
- Treat cracked lips immediately.

What You'll Need

Unfortunately, you probably don't have *everything* you may want to make these balms at home. The details are carefully listed in the recipes but here's a quick rundown on the kinds of things you'll need and their basic uses.

The Base

The base of the balm is made by mixing a combination of the bulky ingredients: carrier oils, butters, and wax.

<u>Sweet almond oil</u> – This oil is a fantastic moisturizer and is rich in vitamins. It has no scent or flavor on its own, so it's ideal for making lip balm.

<u>Grapeseed oil</u> – This oil has anti-aging qualities and it helps to keep your lips smooth and elastic. It's rich in Vitamin E and polyphenols. It smells a little sweet but has no flavor.

<u>Coconut oil</u> – We love coconut oil! It's anti-bacterial, anti-viral, and anti-inflammatory, and it contains vitamins A and C. It even blocks some of the sun's rays. It both smells and tastes of coconut, so you'll keep that in mind when choosing it.

<u>Cocoa butter</u> – Cocoa butter has fatty acids that offer deep moisture for your lips, and it helps prevent wrinkles and fine lines from forming. It also tends to prevent skin irritation. It's vaguely chocolatey, so it's a good choice for some balms more than others.

<u>Shea butter</u> – Shea butter is a natural UV protectant, and it moisturizes and protects the skin. There are many reasons why it's advertised in so many lotions and creams, but we can cut right to the chase and invest in organic shea butter on its own.

<u>Beeswax</u> – Beeswax forms a natural barrier and helps lock in moisture, so it's a very helpful ingredient to have on hand. It's also anti-inflammatory and is known to soothe irritated skin.

As you gain experience, you may find you prefer certain combinations because of the scents or textures that they produce. In general, if your balm comes out too thick, you add a little more oil. If it's too thin, add more butter. If it seems to absorb into the skin and disappear too quickly, a little more wax might be needed.

Additives

Adding things to the base gives you unlimited options for customizing your lip balm.

Essential oils. Using essential oils for scent or flavor are great; just make sure they're 100% pure and used in moderation.

Beetroot, madder, and alkanet powders. You can buy jars or bags of these powders in health food stores or online. They make a great tint for your lip balm.

Food coloring. Go ahead! A drop or two of food coloring can be used in lip balm.

Vitamin E capsules. Easily purchased at any drug or grocery store, these little caplets each contain a few drops of oil that's fantastic for your skin and lips. Feel free to snip a few open and add the contents to any of these balm or gloss recipes.

Containers

There's no need to worry if you don't want to buy little roll-up tubes for your lip balm. They can be found online and at craft stores if you want them, but any small lidded container will do. Be creative! Just be sure to choose something small, (half an ounce is perfect) and that it has a good lid. This reduces the chances of the balm becoming contaminated through long and repeated use.

Now that you have the basics of what's included, let's get started on your DIY lip regimen.

For safety purposes, we also recommend wearing safety glasses to protect your eyes while heating the oils and waxes.

SCRUBS

First things first! Before you apply a mask, balm, or gloss, consider treating your lips to a healthy, exfoliating scrub. Scrubs remove dry and dead skin cells and leave your lips soft and smooth.

Easy Sugar Scrub

A simple scrub that's so simple and easy to make. Use this gentle exfoliant before applying lip balm for amazingly smooth, soft, and luscious lips.

Makes: 0.5 fl.ounce (15 ml)

Ingredients
2 teaspoons granulated sugar or salt
1 teaspoon coconut or sunflower oil
½ teaspoon honey (optional)

Directions
1. Combine the ingredients.
2. Take a pinch of this mixture and rub it gently on your lips to remove rough, dead skin. You may also use a toothbrush to gently loosen dry layers.
3. Leave it on for about a minute, and then wipe it off.
4. Follow with lip balm.
5. Do this not more than once a week.

Vanilla Brown Sugar Lip Scrub

This tasty lip scrub leaves your lips tingling and refreshed.

Makes about ¾ fl.ounce (25 ml)

Ingredients
1 teaspoon coconut oil
½ teaspoon almond oil
2 drops vanilla absolute*
2 teaspoons white sugar
1 tablespoon brown sugar
¼ teaspoon honey

*may sometimes be referred to as an essential oil, but while it is an extract of the vanilla bean, it is technically not an essential oil.

Directions
1. In a small heatproof bowl, melt the coconut oil in the microwave. Add the almond oil and mix well.
2. Add the vanilla, sugars, and honey. Stir to combine.

Gingerbread Lip Scrub

This lip scrub makes a lovely holiday surprise for your friends. The taste is out of this world, and it leaves your lips moisturized and refreshed.

Makes about ¾ fl.ounce (25 ml)

Ingredients
1 ½ tablespoons coconut oil
2 teaspoons honey
2 teaspoons brown sugar
½ teaspoon cinnamon
½ teaspoon ginger
¼ teaspoon nutmeg
Pinch ground cloves

Directions
1. In a small heatproof bowl, melt the coconut oil in the microwave.
2. Add the other ingredients and mix well.

Chocolate Lip Scrub

You can go ahead and lick this off your lips when you're done. We won't judge!

Makes about 2 ½ fl.ounces (75 ml)

Ingredients
3 tablespoons white sugar
1 tablespoon cocoa powder
1 tablespoon olive oil
½ teaspoon vanilla extract
1 teaspoon honey

Directions
1. Combine all the ingredients and mix well.

Citrus Lip Scrub

Citrus oils are anti-microbial, so they help to clean and purify the skin. The fresh scent of this lip scrub is also energizing.

Makes about 1 fl.ounce (35 ml)

Ingredients
1 tablespoon coconut oil
4 teaspoons white sugar
1 drop lemon essential oil
1 drop orange essential oil
1 drop grapefruit essential oil

Directions
1. In a small heatproof bowl, melt the coconut oil in the microwave.
2. Add the other ingredients and mix well.

Vanilla Coffee Lip Scrub

This lip scrub will keep chapped lips moist and smooth in the winter. Plus, it tastes and smells delicious!

Makes about ¼ fl.ounce (7.5 ml) – 1 usage

Ingredients
1 tablespoon coffee grounds, fresh
½ tablespoon jojoba oil
1 teaspoon shea butter
¼ teaspoon Vanilla Absolute

Preparation
1. Mix ingredients together and scoop into an airtight container.

Storage
1. Store in an airtight container for up to 2 weeks. No need to refrigerate.

Directions for Use
1. Rub into dry lips until satisfied.
2. Rinse off and follow with an all-natural lip balm or lip oil.

Oatmeal Lip Scrub

This simple and nourishing lip scrub is as unfussy as it gets. Make it in single batches because it can spoil.

Makes about ¼ fl.ounce (7.5 ml) – 1 usage

Ingredients
1 tablespoon olive oil
1 teaspoon milk powder
2 teaspoons rolled oats

Directions
1. Combine all the ingredients, and apply!

Sugar and Spice Lip Scrub and Plumper

Gently rub off dead layers while smoothing and plumping your lips.

Makes: 1 ½ fl.ounces (45 ml)

Ingredients
1 tablespoon sunflower oil
1 teaspoon sugar
1 teaspoon cinnamon powder

Directions
1. Mix the ingredients together and keep them in a glass container.
2. To use, massage some on your lips and leave it on for 5-10 minutes.
3. Rinse off.

Plumping Coffee Lip Scrub

Invigorate the skin with this delicious coffee scrub!

Makes about 1 fl.ounce (30 ml)

Ingredients
1 tablespoon coconut oil
2 tablespoons brown sugar
2 tablespoons dry coffee grinds

Directions
1. In a small heatproof bowl, melt the coconut oil in the microwave.
2. Add the other ingredients and mix well.

LIP MASKS

Lip masks are simple to make and give the thin and sensitive skin of your lips that extra bit of hydrating support. Most contain vitamins and minerals the skin needs.

If you're looking at commercial products, beware. Many lip masks (like other lip care products) have been found to make false claims. For instance, collagen is not absorbed through the skin, so you can put those products right back on the shelf and keep your money.

Instead, try some of these homemade masks. They contain natural, healthy ingredients that will truly benefit your skin. Most of them will stay on just fine, but if you find your mask softening too much, you can cut a piece of parchment or plastic wrap to press over them.

Honey Avocado Lip Mask

Avocado is a powerhouse of vitamins and minerals that your lips love.

Makes 1 use

Ingredients
1 teaspoon honey
2 teaspoons mashed avocado
2 drops olive oil

Directions
1. Soften the honey and stir in the avocado and olive oil.
2. Apply the mask to the lips and the area around them. Leave it on for 10–15 minutes, and then wipe it off gently with a warm cloth.

Yogurt and Lemon Lip Mask

Give dry and stressed skin a boost with both lactic and citric acid. Follow this mask with a natural balm for a soothing finish.

Makes 1 use

Ingredients
2 teaspoons plain Greek yogurt
½ teaspoon lemon juice
1 drop lemon essential oil

Directions
1. Combine the ingredients and apply them to the lips.
2. Leave the mask on for 5 minutes and then wipe it away with a soft, warm cloth.

Cucumber Green Tea Lip Mask

Combine the soothing properties of cucumber with the antioxidants and tannins in green tea for an excellent lip mask.

Makes 1 use

Ingredients
2 slices cucumber
1 teaspoon honey
½ teaspoon green tea leaves

Directions
1. Peel and seed the cucumber slices. Place the flesh in a bowl and mash it with a fork as much as you can.
2. Stir in the honey and green tea.
3. Apply the mask to the lips.
4. Leave the mask on for 10–15 minutes and then wipe it away with a soft, warm cloth.

Turmeric and Yogurt Lip Mask

Turmeric is increasingly being recognized for its antioxidant and anti-inflammatory capabilities. Try it in this easy lip treatment, especially if you've had too much sun.

Makes 1 use

Ingredients
1 teaspoon Greek yogurt
1 teaspoon honey
½ teaspoon turmeric powder

Directions
1. Combine the ingredients and apply them to the lips.
2. Leave the mask on for 5–10 minutes, and then gently wipe it away.

Aloe Vera Overnight Lip Mask

In this soothing overnight lip treatment, we combine two skincare superheroes: coconut oil and aloe vera! Smooth it on at bedtime and wake up with smooth, healthy lips.

Makes 1 use

Ingredients
½ teaspoon coconut oil
2 teaspoons aloe vera gel
1 drop lavender essential oil

Directions
1. Melt the coconut oil over a double boiler or in the microwave. Let it cool slightly.
2. Add the aloe vera gel and lavender oil, and mix well.
3. Apply at bedtime, and gently wipe it off in the morning.

BALMS

Balms top the list of all the necessary lip care supplies. They moisturize and protect our lips, and many of us are compulsive users. When you make your own using these recipes, that's not a problem at all.

Basic Lip Balm

The best way to protect your lips from the harsh dry elements is to have a nourishing, moisturizing lip balm on hand.

Makes: 1.5 ounces

Ingredients
1 ½ tablespoons beeswax
2 tablespoons cocoa butter
2 tablespoons coconut oil
20 drops of essential oil of choice

Directions
1. Put the beeswax, cocoa butter, and coconut oil into a heatproof glass measuring cup or a mug.
2. Fill a small pot or saucepan with water to reach level of contents of cup or mug (Do not get any water into mixture!) and bring to a simmer.
3. When the contents have melted, turn off the heat but do not take the cup out of the hot water.
4. Stir in the essential oils.
5. Transfer the mixture into containers, or pipette into tubes.
6. Let it cool completely before capping.

Soothing Herbal Lip Balm

This balm soothes the soul as well as the lips. Be sure to use 100% pure essential oil.

Makes about 3 ¾ fl.ounces (110 ml)

Ingredients
4 tablespoons sweet almond oil
2 tablespoons beeswax pellets
1 tablespoon shea butter
10 drops lavender essential oil
Optional: dried lavender flowers or chamomile flowers, crumbled

Directions
1. Prepare containers for the balm. Make sure they are clean and dry and have tight-fitting lids.
2. Heat the oil in a double boiler and stir in the beeswax and shea butter until melted.
3. Add the lavender oil (and flowers if you have them) and stir to combine.
4. Let the mixture cool a little and pour it into jars.

Honey-Coconut Healing Balm

Coconut oil and honey are both excellent moisturizers for the lips. They grab moisture from the air and keep it on the lips. Coconut oil also has antibacterial and antiviral properties that aid in healing, and it offers natural protection from the sun.

Makes: 1 ounce

Ingredients

1 tablespoon grated beeswax or beeswax pastilles
1 tablespoon virgin coconut oil
⅛ teaspoon honey
⅛ teaspoon vitamin E oil
10-15 drops of desired essential oil (try lavender, tea tree oil, or peppermint)

Directions

1. Melt the beeswax in a double boiler.
2. When about half of the beeswax has melted, add the coconut oil and honey.
3. Stir and continue heating until thoroughly melted.
4. Remove it from the heat.
5. Stir in the vitamin E oil and essential oils.
6. Pour the mixture into the prepared containers and let it cool.

Chocolate Mint Lip Balm

This unique balm is sure to be a hit, with its mild chocolate and peppermint flavors and the moisture of cocoa butter and almond oil.

Makes about 2 ½ fl.ounces (75 ml)

Ingredients

2 tablespoons white beeswax pellets
1 tablespoon sweet almond oil
1 tablespoon cocoa butter
1 tablespoon cocoa powder
2–3 drops peppermint oil

Directions

1. Prepare containers for the balm. Make sure they are clean and dry and have tight-fitting lids.
2. Melt the beeswax in the microwave or in a stainless steel bowl over a pot of lightly simmering water. (Don't let the bowl touch the water.)
3. Stir in the almond oil, cocoa butter, cocoa powder, and peppermint. Stir to combine.
4. When it's smooth, dip a dessert spoon in the mixture and let it cool. Check the taste and consistency of what's on the spoon to ensure it's to your liking.
5. If necessary, reheat the mixture to add more flavor. You can also soften balm that is too hard by adding more oil or butter. If the balm is too soft, add more wax.
6. When you're satisfied with the balm, let it cool a little but pour it into the containers before it sets.

Strawberry Lip Balm

Carrot seed oil does not interfere with the taste of this balm, but it does offer some protection from the sun. This is a very popular flavor and it makes a great little present or a colorful addition to a party loot bag. Customize with your favorite flavor of gelatin powder!

Makes about 2 fl.ounces (65 ml)

Ingredients
4 tablespoons coconut oil
1 tablespoon strawberry gelatin mix
2 drops carrot seed essential oil
2 drops of lemon essential oil

Directions
1. Prepare containers for the balm. Make sure they are clean and dry and have tight-fitting lids.
2. Melt the coconut oil in the microwave and add the other ingredients. Mix well.
3. Pour the mixture into the containers and cover.

Honey Lemon Lip Balm

Honey is a natural sweetener and it's antibacterial, too! Enjoy its mild flavor in this pleasant, soothing balm.

Makes about 2 ½ fl.ounces (75 ml)

Ingredients
3 tablespoons beeswax pellets
2 tablespoons coconut oil
4–5 drops lemon essential oil
1 teaspoon honey

Directions
1. Prepare containers for the balm. Make sure they are clean and dry and have tight-fitting lids.
2. Melt the wax and coconut oil in the microwave or double boiler and add the other ingredients. Mix well.
3. When it's smooth, dip a dessert spoon in the mixture and let it cool. Check the taste and consistency of what's on the spoon to ensure it's to your liking.
4. If necessary, reheat the mixture to add more flavor. You can also soften balm that is too hard by adding more coconut oil. If the balm is too soft, add more wax.
5. When you're satisfied with the balm, let it cool a little but pour it into the containers before it sets.

Party Swirl Lip Balm

People go wild for this pretty lip balm, and it smells lovely, too.

Makes about 3 fl.ounces (90 ml)

Ingredients
3 tablespoons beeswax pellets
2 tablespoons coconut oil
1 tablespoon grapeseed oil
3–5 drops orange essential oil
1 teaspoon cherry gelatin powder

Directions
1. Prepare containers for the balm. Make sure they are clean and dry and have tight-fitting lids.
2. Melt the wax and coconut oil in the microwave or double boiler and add the grapeseed oil. Mix well.
3. Spoon out a third of the mixture into a separate bowl. Add the orange oil to the larger portion and stir the cherry gelatin powder into the smaller.
4. Let the mixtures cool slightly, until they are beginning to thicken. Stir again.
5. Pour the orange mixture into the prepared containers, and carefully add the cherry mixture on top. Swirl with a toothpick, and cover.

Lip Plumper Balm

Who wouldn't love to have fuller lips? Well, we'll tell you a secret:
add just a few quick ingredients to a homemade balm recipe,
and you have a safe and easy lip plumper you can use any time.

Makes about 2 ½ fl.ounces (75 ml)

Ingredients
3 tablespoons beeswax pellets
2 tablespoons coconut oil
3–4 drops cinnamon essential oil
Pinch cayenne pepper (optional)
1 teaspoon honey

Directions
1. Prepare containers for the balm. Make sure they are clean and dry and have tight-fitting lids.
2. Melt the wax and coconut oil in the microwave or double boiler and add the other ingredients. Mix well.
3. When it's smooth, dip a dessert spoon in the mixture and let it cool. Check the taste and consistency of what's on the spoon to ensure it's to your liking.
4. If necessary, reheat the mixture to add more flavor. You can also soften balm that is too hard by adding more coconut oil. If the balm is too soft, add more wax.
5. When you're satisfied with the balm, let it cool a little but pour it into the containers before it sets.

Goat's Milk Balm

Goat's milk has been shown to have many benefits for the skin, including maintaining moisture, reducing inflammation, and nourishing with its Vitamin A.

Makes about 3 ½ fl.ounces (110 ml)

Ingredients
2 tablespoons shea butter
2 tablespoons beeswax pellets
2 tablespoons extra virgin olive oil
2 teaspoons Vitamin E oil
2 tablespoons organic goats milk powder

Directions
1. Prepare containers for the balm. Make sure they are clean and dry and have tight-fitting lids.
2. Melt the shea butter and beeswax in a double boiler and then stir in the oils.
3. Stir in the milk powder until smooth.
4. Pour the mixture into the prepared containers and let it set.

Cinnamon White Chocolate Balm

You probably have everything you need to make this tasty and lip-plumping balm.

Makes about 1 fl.ounce (30 ml)

Ingredients
1 tablespoon cocoa butter
1 teaspoon grated beeswax
5 white chocolate chips, chopped
1 teaspoon honey
1 tablespoon grapeseed oil
3 drops cinnamon essential oil

Directions
1. Prepare containers for the balm. Make sure they are clean and dry and have tight-fitting lids.
2. In a double boiler, combine the cocoa butter, beeswax, and chocolate. Heat until they are melted together.
3. Add the honey, grapeseed oil, and cinnamon. Mix well.
4. Pour the mixture into the prepared containers and let it set.

Berry Lemonade Lip Balm

Dried berries are a great way to color and flavor an all-natural lip balm. You can buy freeze dried berries at grocery stores or online. (Here's a hint: we harvested our freeze-dried berries from a box of cereal.)

Makes about 2 ½ fl.ounces (75 ml)

Ingredients
1 tablespoon coconut oil
2 teaspoons beeswax pellets
2 tablespoons crushed freeze-dried berries
1 teaspoon honey
1–2 drops lemon essential oil

Directions
1. Prepare containers for the balm. Make sure they are clean and dry and have tight-fitting lids.
2. In a double boiler, melt the coconut oil and beeswax pellets.
3. Stir in the crushed berries, honey, and oil.
4. Pour the mixture through a strainer into the prepared containers and let it set.

Cinnamon Spice Lip Plumper

Get fuller, plumper, and sexier lips without expensive injections or surgery. The trick is to use mildly irritating ingredients that cause increased blood flow to the lips. The proportion of spices like cinnamon and cayenne causes very mild irritation but, because we all react differently, you'll have to experiment to determine how much will work best for you. This very mild recipe is a good beginner's concoction.

Makes about 0.25 fl.ounces (7.5 ml)

Ingredients
1 tube plain lip balm
½ teaspoon cinnamon oil or powder
¼ - ½ teaspoon cayenne powder, 35 K H.U. (optional)
3-5 drops vanilla flavor oil (optional)

Directions
1. Empty the contents of your lip balm tube (keep the tube for reuse) into a heatproof glass measuring cup or a mug.
2. Fill a small pot or saucepan with water to reach level with the contents of the cup. (Do not get any water into mixture!) and bring it to a simmer.
3. Immerse the measuring cup or mug with the balm in the simmering water (do not boil).
4. Stir, and allow the balm to melt.
5. Add the rest of the ingredients one by one, mixing well after each addition.
6. Transfer the mixture back into the original balm tube or into a container of your choice.

Basic Tinted Balm

Soothing and moisturizing sweet almond and coconut oils, tinted with natural ingredients, will keep your lips looking moist with a hint of color.

Makes: 6 fl. Ounces (180 ml)

Ingredients
¼ cup beeswax
¼ cup sweet almond or coconut oil
¼ cup shea butter
Several drops pure essential oil of choice (such as rose, vanilla, or lavender)
1 teaspoon beetroot powder or cocoa powder (or a combination), for color

Directions
1. Put the beeswax in a heatproof glass measuring cup, or a mug.
2. Fill a small pot or saucepan with water to reach the level of the contents of the mug (Do not get any water into the mixture!) and bring it to a simmer.
3. Immerse the measuring cup or mug with the balm in the simmering water (do not boil).
4. Stir and allow the beeswax to melt.
5. When half of the beeswax has melted, add the sweet almond oil and shea butter. Allow everything to melt.
6. Stir with a stainless steel spoon. To test for consistency, lift a small amount with the spoon and allow it to cool. Adjust the consistency by adding more beeswax (to thicken) or more oil (to thin), as needed.

Basic Fruit Tinted Lip Balm

You can use your favorite fruit to make this simple and easy to make lip balm for a solid lip moisturizer and protector.

Makes about 1 fl.ounce (30 ml)

Ingredients
2 tablespoons coconut oil
1 teaspoon beeswax or ¾ teaspoon soy wax
½ teaspoon dried and powdered berries or fruit (berries work best; raspberries give a pink hue, blackberries a dark mauve, blueberries more purple, peach light yellow)
Ice cubes for testing

Directions
1. Put your wax and coconut oil in the top pot or bowl of the double boiler or in the microwavable dish. Melt in the double boiler, or heat for 30 seconds in the microwave, take it out with an oven mitt, stir it, and put it back in for 15-second bursts until it is completely melted. If there are only seed-sized pieces not melted, stirring the hot liquid will allow them to melt down without excessive heating.

2. Add your finely powdered berries or fruit and stir the mixture well. Then take out the ice cube. Put it on a piece of paper or paper towel and drip a small drop of the mixture onto the ice cube. Swipe it off with your finger and rub it on your lips. If it is too greasy, it needs more wax. If it is too stiff, it needs more coconut oil. Once you have the right consistency, carefully pour the liquid into the small container. You may need to re-stir with a toothpick occasionally if the fruit begins to settle. Let it cool and put the lid on. This balm should hold up well in average temperatures but could begin to melt above 85º F.

GLOSSES AND TINTS

If you're looking for shine as well as a healthy lip treatment, that's no problem. These recipes tend to use more oil than wax or butters, so the result is shinier and you might want to buy tubes to hold the mixture. Even if you make that investment, the finished gloss is better for you and much less expensive than similar commercial products.

Basic Natural Lip Gloss

This is the easiest recipe to make your own all-natural lip gloss.

Makes about ¾ fl.ounces (22 ml)

Ingredients
1 teaspoon beeswax or ¾ tablespoon soy wax
4 teaspoons coconut oil
2 teaspoons jojoba, olive oil, grape seed, or hemp oil
4 drops essential oil of your choice (optional)

Directions
1. Place the coconut oils and jojoba (or others), and wax into the top of a double boiler or into your microwavable-safe dish. Stir until melted. For the microwave, heat at 30 seconds, stir, and then use 15-second bursts until the wax is melted. Stir the mixture until all of the melted waxes and oils are incorporated.
2. If you would like to add essential oils, add it in now and whisk until it is thoroughly mixed.
3. Pour the gloss into the container and allow to cool. This mixture can liquefy in hot environments, so make sure to seal the container well before putting it in your purse.

Sinus Relief Lip Gloss

Whip up a batch of this soothing lip gloss when the cold season hits! Its gentle fumes will help clear a stuffy nose.

Makes about 3 ½ fl.ounces (110 ml)

Ingredients
2 tablespoons beeswax pellets
2 tablespoons almond oil
2 tablespoons coconut oil
1 tablespoon olive oil
1 tablespoon honey
4 drops peppermint oil
4 drops eucalyptus oil

Directions
1. Prepare containers for the lip gloss, either tubs or tubes. Make sure they are clean and dry and have tight-fitting lids.
2. Boil 2 inches of water in a saucepan.
3. Place the beeswax, almond oil, coconut oil, and olive oil in a mason jar and place it in the water.
4. Stirring from time to time, heat the jar until everything is melted.
5. Stir in the honey and essential oils. When it's cool enough, pour it into the jars or tubes and seal.

Candy Lip Gloss

Little girls love to dress up, and sometimes that might mean wearing makeup. Good news! This easy homemade lip gloss tastes great and is 100% safe for your little ones.

Makes about 1 ¾ fl.ounces (50 ml)

Ingredients

1 packet unsweetened powdered drink mix
1 teaspoon hot water
2 tablespoons coconut oil
1 tablespoon shea butter
1 teaspoon honey

Directions

1. Prepare containers for the gloss.
2. In a small bowl, add the hot water to the drink mix and stir until the mixture is dissolved. Set aside.
3. In a microwave-safe dish, melt the coconut oil and shea butter. Stir in the honey.
4. Add a few drops of the dissolved drink mix until you're satisfied with the color and flavor of the mixture.
5. Pour the gloss into the containers and seal.

Healthy Lip Tint

Sometimes you want a little color on your lips. Put away that commercial lipstick! Try this easy peasy recipe, made of things that are good for you. You can use it on your cheeks, too.

Makes about 1 fl.ounce (30 ml)

Ingredients
1 tablespoon sweet almond oil OR shea butter
1 tablespoon beet powder (or to your liking)
2 drops essential oil of your choice for scent (optional, we love lavender)

Directions
1. Prepare containers for the gloss.
2. In a small bowl over a double boiler, warm the oil or butter.
3. Stir in the beet powder until it is well combined. You can add more or less color, depending on the shade you want.
4. If there is still sediment in the gloss, you can choose to strain it through a piece of muslin or cheesecloth.
5. Add the essential oil, if using.
6. Pour the lip tint into the prepared container(s).

Candy Corn Lip Gloss

If you're a fan of candy corn, you'll love this easy and tasty gloss.

Makes about 2 ½ fl.ounces (80 ml)

Ingredients
2 tablespoons coconut oil
1 tablespoon sweet almond oil
8 candy corns, grated
1 teaspoon grated beeswax
Optional: orange food coloring

Directions
1. Prepare containers for the gloss.
2. In a small, microwave-safe bowl, combine all the ingredients EXCEPT the food coloring.
3. Place the dish in the microwave and heat it on 50%, stirring every 10 seconds until everything is combined.
4. Add the color, if using.
5. Pour the gloss into the containers and seal.

Custom Tinted Gloss

We love this recipe! The beeswax gives the gloss some staying power, while also hydrating and protecting the lips. It's well worth investing in madder and alkanet powders so you can experiment and create your own best shade.

Makes about 2 fl.ounces (60 ml)

Ingredients
1 ½ ounces sweet almond oil
About ¾ teaspoons total colored powders, in combination of madder, alkanet, cocoa
½ ounce beeswax pellets
1 ounce shea or cocoa butter

Directions
1. Prepare containers for the gloss.
2. In a small bowl over a double boiler, warm the almond oil.
3. Stir in the combination of powders, watching as you go to see the shade you're creating.
4. Strain the oil into a bottle.
5. Melt the beeswax and shea or cocoa butter in a double boiler. Stir in the infused oil and mix well.
6. Carefully pour the balm into the prepared container(s) and let it set.

HEALTHY LIPSTICKS

Lipsticks make the lips appear fuller and more attractive, boosting the wearer's confidence level about her appearance. A makeup kit is never complete without lipstick.

Homemade Lipstick

The rich coconut oil and cocoa butter in this recipe keep your lips soft and hydrated in your own concocted color using mica powder. Mica powder is a safe and natural coloring agent that reflects light, making your lips look smooth and shimmery.

Makes 4 fl. Ounces (120 ml)

Ingredients
3 tablespoons coconut oil
3 tablespoons cocoa butter
3 tablespoons beeswax
10 drops essential oil of choice (vanilla, grapefruit, rose, orange, etc.)
1 teaspoon mica powder (in a shade or combination of shades of your choice)

Directions
1. Melt the coconut oil, cocoa butter, and beeswax in a double boiler.
2. When fully melted, stir in the essential oils and mica powder. Mix well. Turn off the heat, but leave the mixture in the double boiler to keep it liquid.
3. To test the color and consistency, use a toothpick to pick up a small amount. Allow it to cool and test it on your lips. You may need to add a little more melted beeswax to make it harder, or more mica powder for more color.
4. Pour the mixture into prepared containers. If you are using tubes, use a pipette to transfer the mixture.
5. Allow the lipstick to cool before placing caps.

Natural Lipstick

An easy to make lipstick with a natural tint of cocoa powder.

Makes 2 fl. ounces (60 ml)

Ingredients
2 teaspoons beeswax
2 teaspoons shea butter
4 teaspoons sweet almond oil
2 teaspoons coconut oil
4 drops any essential oil
A pinch cocoa powder

Preparation
1. Add the shea butter and beeswax to a double boiler and melt them.
2. Add the oils and cocoa powder and remove from heat.
3. Add the essential oil and mix well.
4. Store in a lipstick tube.

Basic Red Lipstick

This easy to prepare lipstick has only 3 ingredients and you can make ir as dark as you want it.

Makes 1 fl. Ounce (30 ml)

Ingredients
1 tablespoon olive oil
1 tablespoon beeswax
1 beetroot, dried and grated

Preparation
1. Melt the beeswax and olive oil in a double boiler.
2. Slowly add the grated beetroot to the mixture as you keep stirring.
3.   Allow the lipstick to cool and then transfer to a container.

Color and Plump Lipstick

A two-in-one lipstick that colors and gently plumps your lips. Its moisturizing ingredients ensure that your lips are always in great condition.

Makes: 4 fl. Ounces (120 ml)

Ingredients
3 tablespoons sweet almond oil
3 tablespoons cocoa butter
3 tablespoons beeswax
1 drop cinnamon oil
1 drop ginger oil
3-5 drops peppermint essential oil
1 drop clove oil (optional)
1 teaspoon mica powder (in a shade or combination of shades of your choice)

Directions
1. Melt the almond oil, cocoa butter, and beeswax in a double boiler.
2. When they are fully melted, stir in the essential oils and mica powder. Mix well. Turn off the heat, but leave the mixture in the double boiler to keep liquid.
3. To test the color and consistency, use a toothpick to pick up a small amount. Allow it to cool and test it on your lips. You may need to add a little more melted beeswax to make it harder, or more mica powder for more color.
4. Pour the mixture into prepared containers. If you are using tubes, use a pipette to transfer the mixture.

NATURAL REMEDIES FOR LIPS

Natural Remedies for Chapped, Dry, and Split Lips

Factors that can cause chapped lips include:

- Smoking
- Drinking
- Excessive licking of lips
- Sun exposure
- Dehydration
- Allergy
- Harsh weather

Split lips can be caused by harsh weather conditions, lip injuries, excessive licking of the lips, and dryness.

Given below are the best natural remedies to heal chapped and split lips:

1) Honey

The moisturizing and antibacterial properties of honey help to heal lips fast. Honey also retains moisture.

Apply a drop or two of honey to the lips. Repeat it several times a day until your lips improve.

2) Honey and Vaseline

Vaseline nourishes the lips and retains moisture. Using it along with honey can be very effective in treating chapped and split lips.

Apply honey to your lips, then apply Vaseline on top of the honey. Wipe off with a damp cloth after 15 minutes.

3) Coconut Oil

The moisturizing and lubricating properties of coconut oil help to keep your lips soft, prevent dryness, and heal cracks.

Add one to two drops of tea tree oil to two drops of coconut oil. Apply the mixture to your lips and leave it to be absorbed.

4) Cucumber

Cucumber hydrates the lips and prevents dryness.

Rub a cucumber slice on your lips for 1 minute. Rinse off after 10 minutes. Alternately, you can apply cucumber paste on your lips.

5) Butter

The essential fatty acids in butter hydrate the skin.

Apply some butter on your lips and massage gently. Leave it overnight.

6) Aloe Vera

Aloe vera has moisturizing properties. It keeps the lips moisturized and heals chapped lips.

Extract some gel from an aloe vera leaf. Apply the gel on your lips and massage gently. Leave it overnight.

7) Lemon Juice and Honey

Lemon exfoliates and bleaches the lips. Honey keeps the lips moisturized.

Mix together a teaspoon each of lemon juice and honey. Apply to your lips. Rinse after 10 to 15 minutes.

Natural Remedies for Cold Sores on Lips

Cold sores, an infectious condition, can show up in any part of the body, but they generally occur on the lips, nose, cheeks and fingers. Though not serious, they can be painful. They can also be cured using natural remedies.

1) Lemon Balm
Lemon balm destroys the virus that causes cold sores.

Apply lemon balm to the affected area. Wash off after half an hour. Repeat once a day until the condition is cured.

2) Aloe Vera
Aloe vera is a potent antioxidant that fights infections and promotes healing.

Extract some gel from an aloe vera leaf and apply it to the sore. Leave it overnight.

3) Vanilla Oil
Vanilla oil possesses anti-inflammatory properties that cure infection and promote healing.

Dip a cotton ball in vanilla oil and apply it to the affected area. Wash off after a few minutes. Repeat until pain subsides and condition improves.

4) Garlic
The enzymes in garlic act as antiviral and antibacterial agents and aid in healing cold sores.

Crush a clove of garlic. Apply the crushed garlic to the cold sore. Rinse off after 10 minutes. Repeat 5 to 6 times a day.

5) Tea Tree Oil

The antiviral properties of tea tree oil support healing of cold sores.

Dilute a few drops of tea tree oil in water. Dip a small cotton ball in the diluted solution and apply it to the affected area. Leave it to dry. Repeat twice daily until symptoms improve.

Tips to Prevent Cold Sores

- Increase vitamin C intake.
- Increase intake of foods rich in zinc.
- Avoid stress triggers. Stress can raise the frequency of cold sores when the immune function is low.
- Stay away from spicy foods.
- Apply sunscreen.

Home Remedies to Lighten Dark Lips

The concerns about lips can be never-ending if you don't follow a healthy lifestyle. Cold sores, dry lips and dark lips can all be caused by poor immune system function due to an unhealthy lifestyle. Dark lips can result from dryness, excessive intake of coffee and tea, smoking, sun exposure, and reactions to certain cosmetics. Dark lips can be lightened using the following natural remedies.

1) Lemon Juice

Lemon contains vitamin C, which lightens dark lips. Lemon removes dead cells as well.

Add a teaspoon of sugar to the juice of half a lemon. Mix, apply to your lips and massage gently. Leave for about 15 minutes. Rinse off with water.

2) Coconut Oil

The essential fatty acids in coconut oil keep the lips hydrated, thereby lightening the lips.

Take two drops of coconut oil and apply it to your lips. Massage gently. Leave it on overnight.

3) Honey

Honey is a natural moisturizer. It also nourishes the lips and lightens dark lips.

Take some honey and apply it to your lips. Massage for a minute. Wash off after 15 to 20 minutes. You can also apply honey at night and leave it overnight.

4) Beetroot

Beetroot works great to remove a tan, and it's also effective for lightening dark lips.

Gently rub a slice of beetroot on your lips for a minute or two. Let it remain for about 15 minutes before washing it off.

5) Aloe Vera

The aloesin in aloe vera checks skin pigmentation and lightens the lips. It also nourishes the lips.

Apply aloe vera gel on the lips. Let it air dry before rinsing it off.

6) Baking Soda

Baking soda exfoliates the skin. Removal of dead cells helps to return the lips to their original color.

Add some water to baking soda to make a thick paste. Apply it to the lips. Scrub for a couple of minutes. Wash off and apply some coconut oil to your lips.

ALSO BY JOSEPHINE SIMON

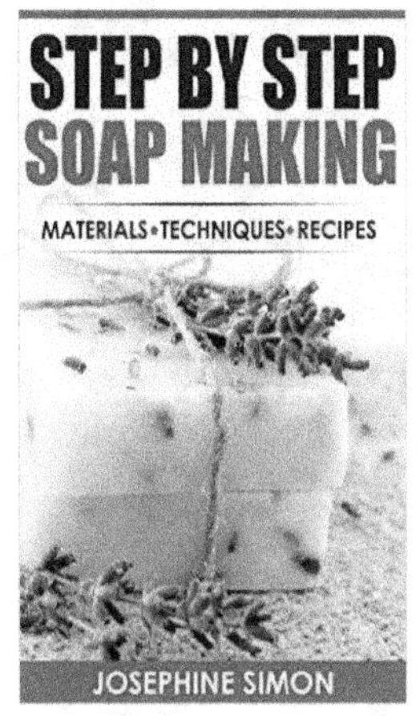

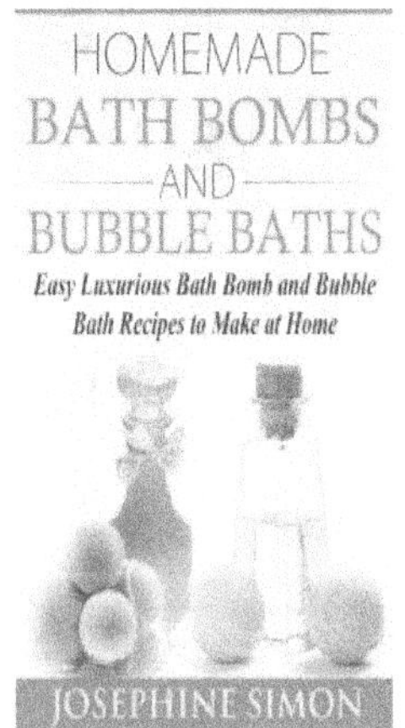

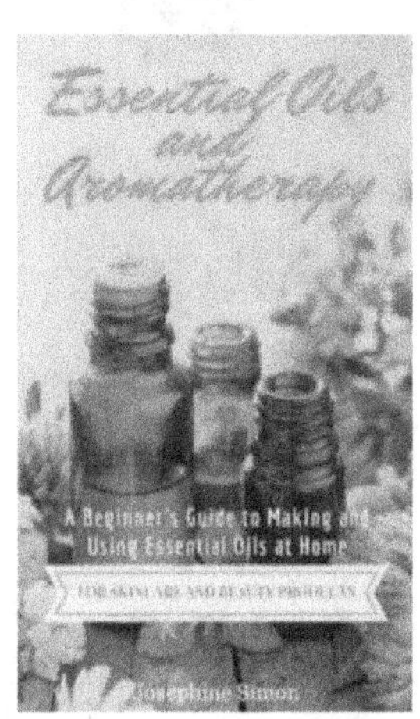

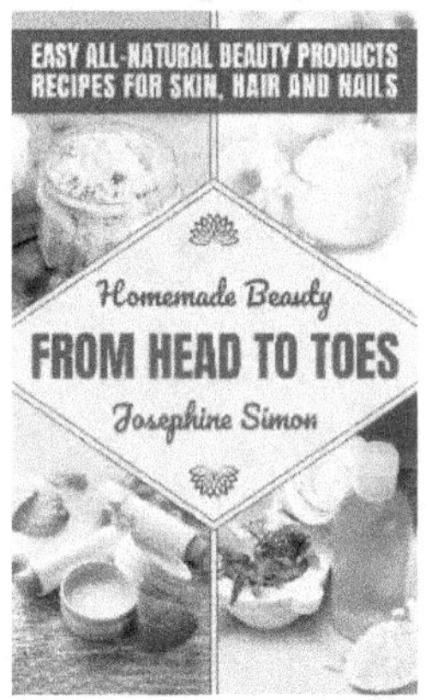

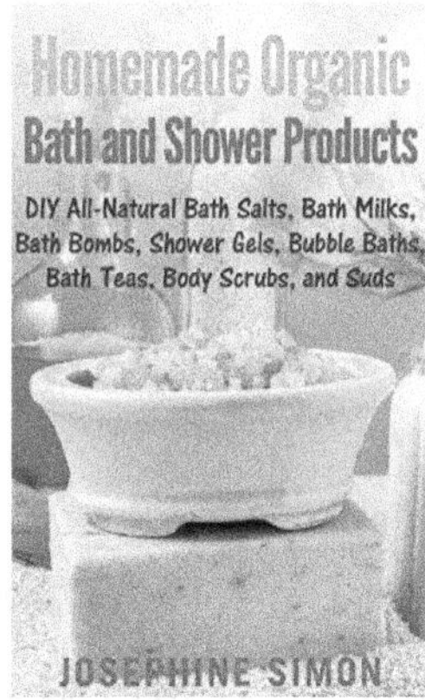

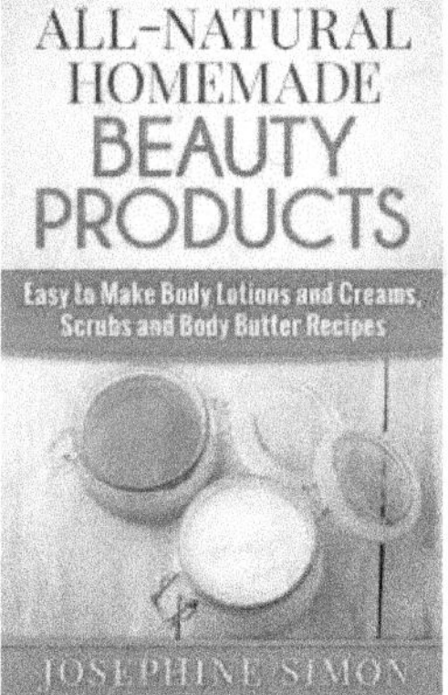

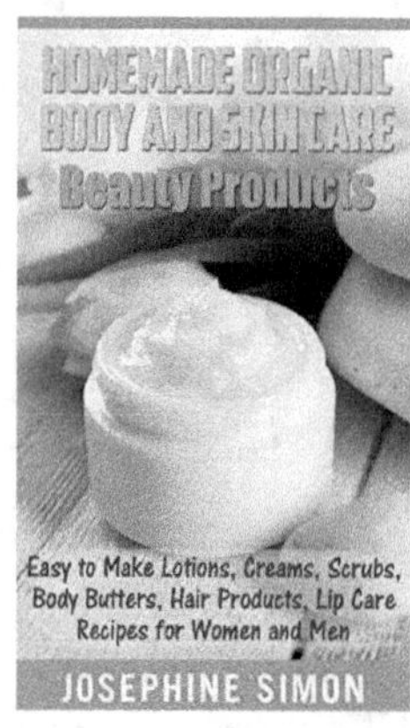

HOMEMADE ORGANIC
BODY AND SKIN CARE
Beauty Products
Easy to Make Lotions, Creams, Scrubs,
Body Butters, Hair Products, Lip Care
Recipes for Women and Men
JOSEPHINE SIMON

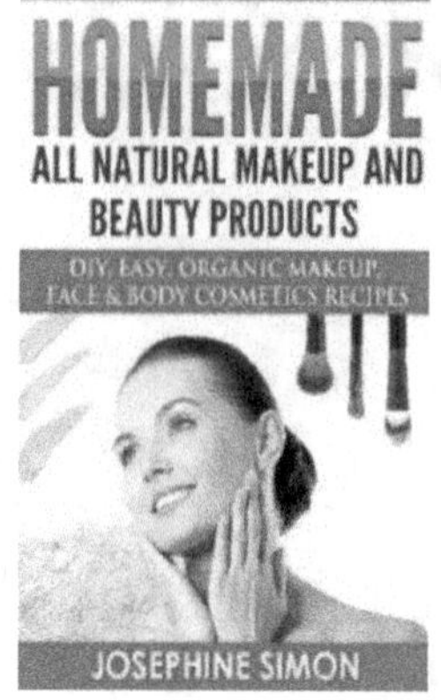

HOMEMADE
ALL NATURAL MAKEUP AND
BEAUTY PRODUCTS
DIY, EASY, ORGANIC MAKEUP,
FACE & BODY COSMETICS RECIPES
JOSEPHINE SIMON

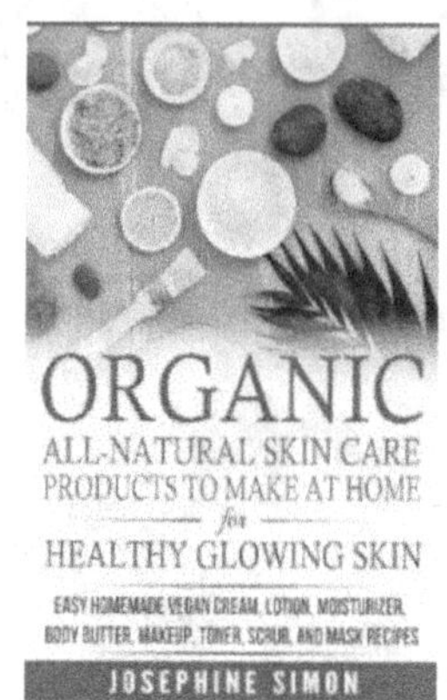

ORGANIC
ALL-NATURAL SKIN CARE
PRODUCTS TO MAKE AT HOME
for
HEALTHY GLOWING SKIN
EASY HOMEMADE VEGAN CREAM, LOTION, MOISTURIZER,
BODY BUTTER, MAKEUP, TONER, SCRUB, AND MASK RECIPES
JOSEPHINE SIMON

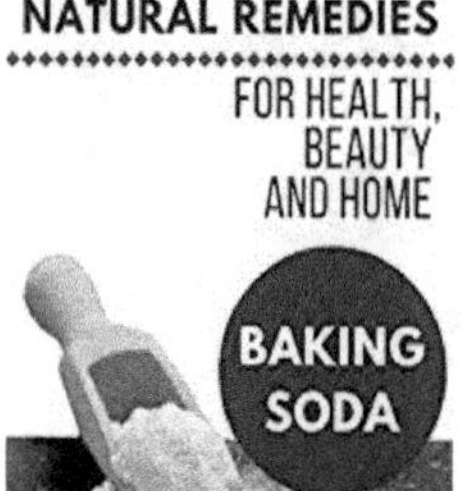

NATURAL REMEDIES
FOR HEALTH,
BEAUTY
AND HOME
BAKING
SODA
JOSEPHINE SIMON

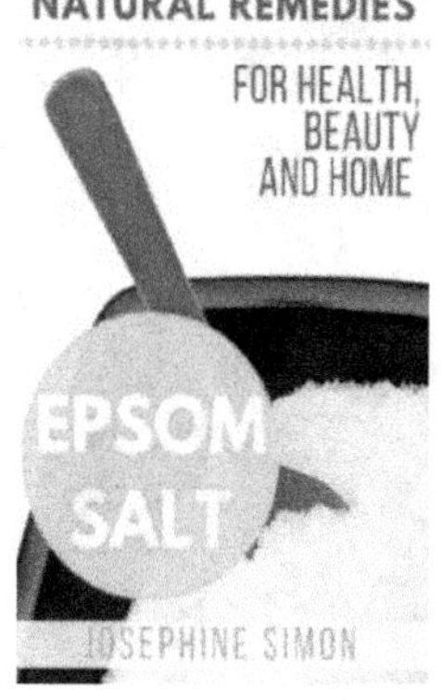

NATURAL REMEDIES
FOR HEALTH,
BEAUTY
AND HOME
EPSOM
SALT
JOSEPHINE SIMON

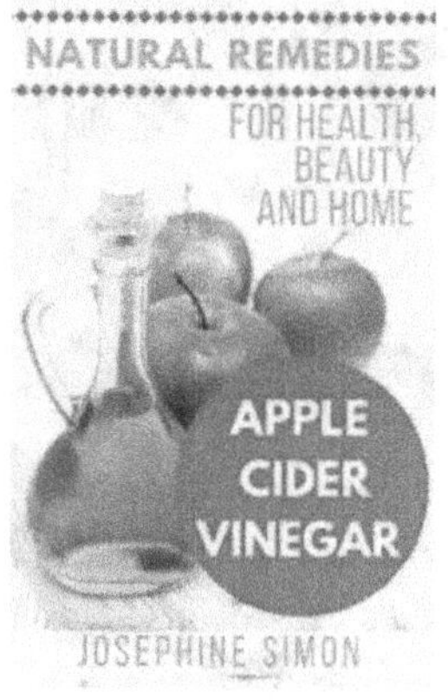

NATURAL REMEDIES
FOR HEALTH,
BEAUTY
AND HOME
APPLE
CIDER
VINEGAR
JOSEPHINE SIMON

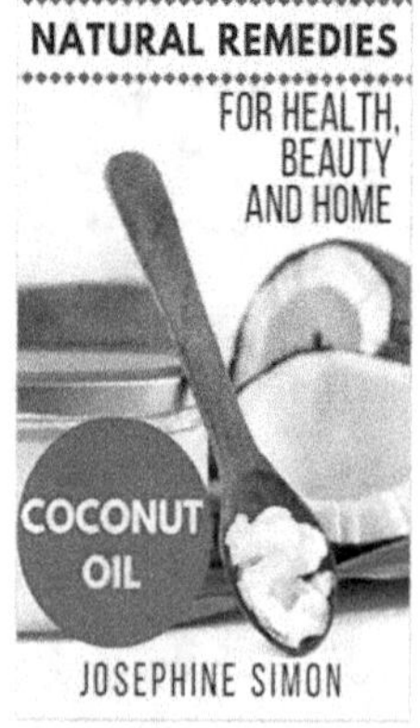

NATURAL REMEDIES
FOR HEALTH,
BEAUTY
AND HOME
COCONUT
OIL
JOSEPHINE SIMON

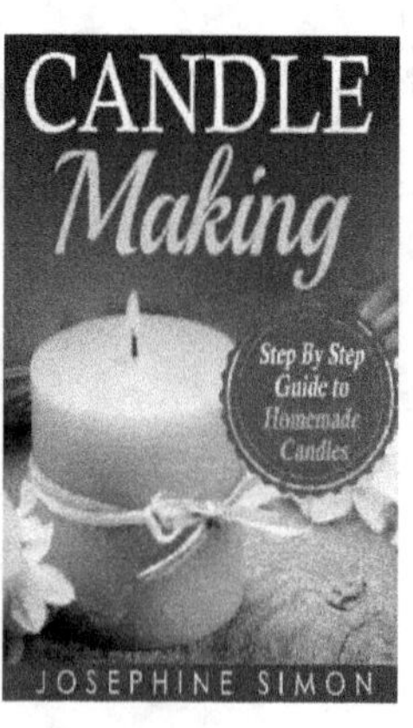

CANDLE
Making
Step By Step
Guide to
Homemade
Candles
JOSEPHINE SIMON